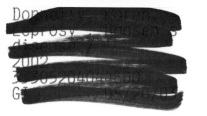

KAREN DONNELLY

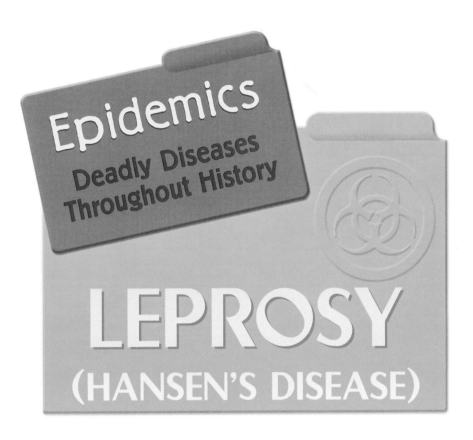

Epidemics
Deadly Diseases
Throughout History

LEPROSY
(HANSEN'S DISEASE)

The Rosen Publishing Group, Inc.
New York

To my family, Colleen, Cathy, and David.

Published in 2002 by The Rosen Publishing Group, Inc.
29 East 21st Street, New York, NY 10010

Library of Congress Cataloging-in-Publication Data

Donnelly, Karen.
Leprosy (Hansen's disease) / by Karen Donnelly. — 1st ed.
p. cm. — (Epidemics)
Includes bibliographical references and index.
Summary: Presents information about leprosy from a historical perspective, including its spread, its treatment, and its future.
ISBN 0-8239-3498-5
1. Leprosy—Juvenile literature. [1. Leprosy. 2. Diseases.]
I. Title: Hansen's disease. II. Title. III. Series.
RC154 .D66 2001
616.9'98—dc21

                                                    2001003051

Cover image: Electron micrograph of the *Mycobacterium leprae* bacteria, which causes leprosy.

Manufactured in the United States of America

CONTENTS

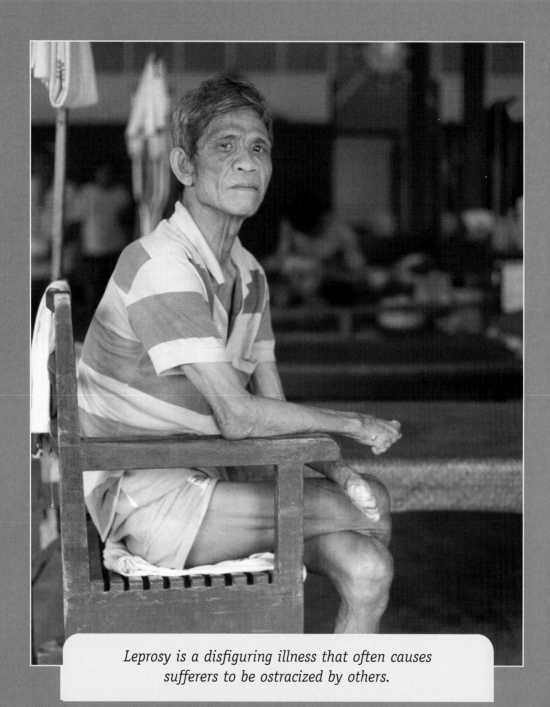

Leprosy is a disfiguring illness that often causes sufferers to be ostracized by others.

INTRODUCTION

Throughout history, people have lived in cities, urban areas where traders gathered to sell their wares and soldiers returned from wars. Neighbors met on the street and in each other's homes. The aristocracy could not avoid contact with peasants. Every day, people of all kinds mixed together.

Within this mix, disease spread more easily than it did in rural areas. The life expectancy of the citizens of ancient Rome, for example, was much shorter than that of people living in the far reaches of the Roman Empire. Only about one-third of city-dwelling Romans lived to be thirty years of age. In outlying areas, 70 percent of the population reached thirty. Some 15 percent lived to be eighty years of age.

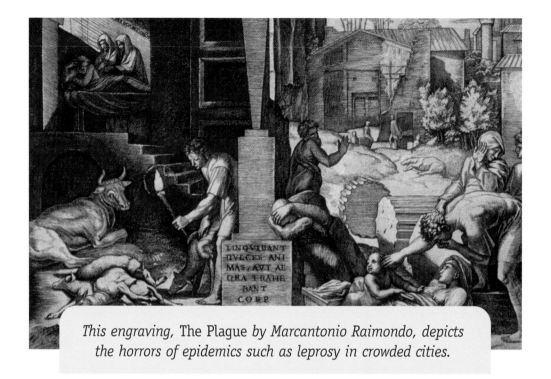

This engraving, The Plague *by Marcantonio Raimondo, depicts the horrors of epidemics such as leprosy in crowded cities.*

The close human contact created by living conditions in the city made the spread of infectious diseases—diseases that can be "caught"—nearly impossible to control. Houses were built right next to each other. Rats ran freely from home to home, carrying fleas, ticks, and other insects that could cause illness. People crowded into small rooms, where a cough or a sneeze sent bacteria (microorganisms that cause sickness) through the air from one person to another.

During the Middle Ages (the fifth century to the fifteenth century) in Europe, disease terrorized people. No one knew what caused bubonic plague, tuberculosis, or leprosy. Some people believed that God sent the disease to punish people for their sins.

Others wondered if Satan was at work. Sometimes, groups of innocent people were killed by angry mobs who blamed them for causing disease.

The terror continued until the late seventeenth century, when the microscope was invented. Before that, no one knew that bacteria existed. These tiny organisms cannot be seen with the naked eye. Even when Norwegian biologist Gerhard Henrick Armauer Hansen first discovered in 1873 the bacteria that cause leprosy, he had difficulty convincing people that something so small could result in such a horrible disease. However, his discovery led to further research and eventually to a cure. Today, leprosy is also called Hansen's disease in his honor.

Through scientific advances, researchers have now discovered the bacteria or viruses that cause many infectious diseases. Drugs have been developed to treat and cure these diseases. For many today, vaccines can prevent infection.

But new diseases still appear, no less terrifying than the plagues of the Middle Ages. AIDS, which destroys the body's immune system—its ability to fight off infection—has killed millions around the world. AIDS can now be better controlled by treatment with drugs, although there is no cure. But in poorer countries, especially those in Africa, the drugs are not widely available. People continue to die by the thousands.

Like AIDS, today leprosy can be controlled by drugs. But in poor countries, people still are not able to get the care they need. The same conditions of over-crowding, malnutrition, and poor sanitation that caused the spread of leprosy in cities in the Middle Ages still exist today in places like India and Brazil.

1

WHAT IS LEPROSY?

Leprosy is an infectious disease caused by bacteria called *Mycobacterium leprae* that hide in the coolest areas of the body. Leprosy can strike at any age but most often afflicts those between ten and twenty years of age. Cases have been seen in infants as young as two and a half months. Infection after age seventy is not uncommon. Men are twice as likely as women to get leprosy.

Types of Leprosy

The simplest form of leprosy, the indeterminate type, primarily affects the skin, causing swollen, reddish patches while the body's immune system tries to fight off the disease. For many people, this battle succeeds. The red patches disappear when the fight has been won and the bacteria are gone. If the bacteria are able to overpower the body's immune system, however, the germs grow and their

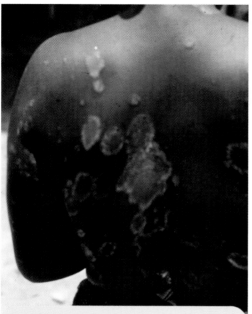

This woman's leprosy has caused swollen, reddish patches, or lesions, on the skin of her back.

numbers increase, and the leprosy becomes the lepromatous type, the tuberculoid type, or the borderline type, which is somewhere in between.

With the lepromatous type, skin on the face and around the nose "thickens," making the face appear swollen. If lepromatous leprosy is not treated, the cartilage (the hard tissue) around the nose can be destroyed, and the nose will look like it has caved in.

Leprosy can also affect the nerves that control the sweat glands and the sebaceous glands, which are the glands that keep skin moist. This can cause hair loss, especially loss of eyebrows. Drying skin cracks, causing open sores that can become infected.

Another form of leprosy, the tuberculoid type, affects the nerves nearest the outside of the body. One of the jobs of these nerves is to tell the brain when a part of the body, like the hands or feet, is in pain. When the nerves have been damaged by leprosy, they are unable to send the message of pain to the brain. Fingers, hands, toes, and feet become numb. Sometimes, leprosy keeps the nerve cells of the eye from telling the brain that dust is painfully itchy. This can cause damage that may lead to blindness. The tuberculoid type of leprosy also causes skin sores. But because the nerve cells do not tell the brain that these sores are painful, they may go untreated and worsen. The diseased cells eat away at healthy tissue, destroying fingers and toes.

Serious injuries often happen to people with leprosy because they do not realize that they are in danger. A woman may be holding her hand so near a flame that she is getting badly burned. But because she does not feel pain, her brain will not tell her to pull her hand away. When trying to lift a rock, a man may drop it on his foot, smashing his toe. He may not feel the intense pain this injury should cause. Instead, he could continue to walk

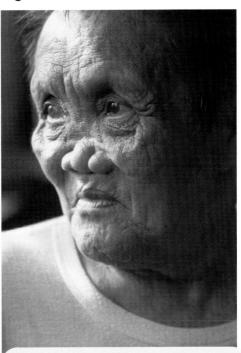

If leprosy is not treated, the cartilage in the nose can be destroyed, and the nose will look like it has collapsed.

for days without treatment. Leprosy has shut off the pain signal to the brain. These injuries can get worse, become infected, and lead to serious disabilities.

Sometimes, the hands and feet of leprosy victims must be amputated, or removed, because they have been hurt very badly by repeated injuries. Many believe leprosy causes toes, fingers, and even noses to fall off. But this is not true. Leprosy does not cause parts of the body to fall off.

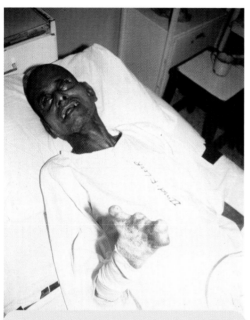

Leprosy does not cause body parts to fall off. However, sometimes they are so injured, they must be amputated.

Leprosy can also affect motor nerves, the nerves that the brain uses to tell the hands, feet, and even eyelids to move. People with leprosy may be unable to close their eyes. Blindness can result because the eyes become dry or damaged without the protection of the eyelids. Also, hands or feet hang loosely in a condition called dropped foot or dropped wrist. Or, the hand may "freeze" in a position that looks like a claw.

How Leprosy Is Contracted

Although scientists have discovered the *Mycobacterium leprae* (known as *M. leprae*) bacteria that cause leprosy, they still do not know how people get it. Daniel C. Danielssen, a nineteenth-century Norwegian scientist, observed that the ability to fight off the disease seemed to run in families. He also noticed that he and his assistants did not get leprosy even though they worked very closely with people who had it. He thought this meant that leprosy was not a contagious disease. Instead, he believed the disease was inherited and children got it because their parents or other relatives had it.

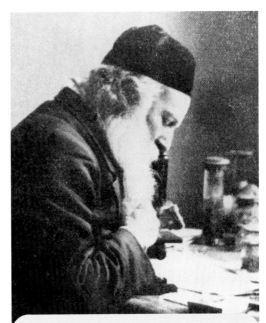

Daniel C. Danielssen pioneered the diagnosis and treatment of leprosy, but thought the disease was not contagious.

Danielssen tried an experiment to prove his theory. He and four of his assistants injected themselves with leprosy cells that they had taken from their patients. As he had predicted, Danielssen and his

600 BC
The first full accounts of leprosy are found in Indian writings.

1340s
The Black Plague ravishes Europe, wiping out leprosy as well.

1866
The first leprosy victims arrive at Kalaupapa leprosy settlement on the Hawaiian island of Molokai.

1095–1272
The Crusades are responsible for the spread of leprosy throughout Europe and the Middle East.

assistants did not get leprosy. At the time, Danielssen was believed to know more about leprosy than other scientists. Most of them accepted his "proof" that leprosy was not contagious.

Today, scientists believe that leprosy is contagious. It is likely, though, that most people, as much as 90 percent of the population, are naturally immune to leprosy. Their bodies are able to fight off the leprosy bacteria and they do not get sick. This natural immunity may be hereditary. Scientists believe, however, that people who are naturally immune may still be able to carry the bacteria and pass the bacteria to other people. Even though they do not get sick themselves, they can make other people sick.

1873	1941	1982
Mycobacterium leprae is discovered by Dr. Armauer Hansen.	The Miracle at Carville: Dr. Guy Faget discovers treatment for leprosy.	Multidrug therapy becomes the treatment recognized and used by the World Health Organization.

1894	2000
Leprosy patients are taken by barge to Carville, an abandoned plantation in Louisiana.	Around the world, leprosy is reduced by 86 percent.

People who have leprosy seem to have contracted it from close contact with others who are infected. But no one knows exactly how the disease is passed. One theory suggests that touching the skin of an infected person is all it takes. Scientists have not ruled out the possibility that insects, especially houseflies, could carry the bacteria. Houseflies can carry as many as six million bacteria on their feet. If these insects walk on infected tissue, like open sores, then they will take the leprosy bacteria with them.

It is possible that the bacteria are breathed in from an infected person who has coughed or sneezed nearby. The most widely accepted theory is that tiny droplets from the nose of an infected person carry the bacteria to someone else. Scientists believe that these bacteria can live outside the body and ride around on clothing for at least thirty-six hours. Under hot, humid conditions, they can live for several days, making it very difficult to tell where the germs came from.

Researchers have trouble finding out how people get leprosy because it is so hard to tell when or where they got it. The leprosy bacteria can lie dormant, as if they were sleeping, and hide inside the body. They can "sleep" for a few weeks or as long as twenty years before causing symptoms. So much time passes that victims cannot remember exactly how they could have contracted the disease.

Although leprosy rarely causes death, it weakens the immune system, making infection by other diseases, like pneumonia, more likely. And the disabilities it causes can be dreadful. Perhaps the most damaging effects are those caused by ignorance and fear. People in some cultures still believe that victims of leprosy have done something to deserve their disease. They are still treated as outcasts. Today, most doctors under-stand that leprosy is totally curable. They are working to wipe it out.

2

LEPROSY IN HISTORY

No one knows for sure when the leprosy bacteria first appeared. Sacred writings in India as far back as 1400 BC referred to *kushtha*, which may have meant leprosy. However, more likely, this word included a whole range of skin diseases. Similarly, the Hebrew word *tzara'ath*, found in the Old Testament, probably did not specifically refer to leprosy as we know it today. Even the Greek word *lepra* in the New Testament, from which leprosy gets its name, included more common skin conditions, like psoriasis.

In the Middle Ages, however, biblical references were used to support the practice of isolating victims of leprosy, who were thought to be cursed by God. In the Old Testament Book of Numbers, God tells Moses to send away anyone who has an infectious skin disease because they are "defiled," or unclean. In 2 Chronicles, King Uzziah of Judah is afflicted with leprosy as punishment for his pride

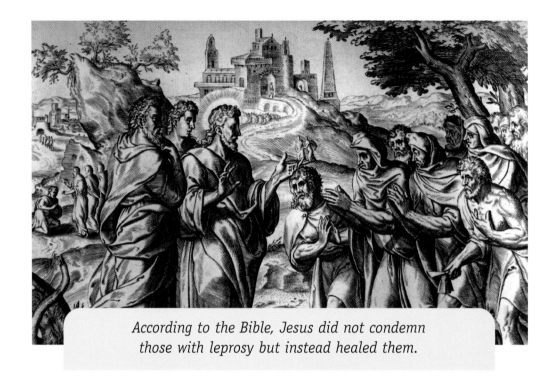

According to the Bible, Jesus did not condemn those with leprosy but instead healed them.

and unfaithfulness. He is banned from the temple and forced to give up the throne to his son. In the New Testament, Jesus cures a leper by making him "clean." Later, Christian societies would use these stories as proof that victims of leprosy were sinners and deserved their disease.

Christian writings were not the first evidence of leprosy. As early as the fifth century BC, a disease like leprosy was described in Indian and Chinese medical writings. Archaeologists have discovered mummies in Egypt dating back to the second century BC that show signs of leprosy. The earliest description of leprosy in the West can be found in the *Canon of Medicine*, written by tenth-century Persian physician Avicenna.

The Spread of Leprosy

Like many other diseases, leprosy was spread by world exploration and war. Alexander the Great's campaign to India in 327 BC may have brought leprosy to Alexandria, Egypt. Most scholars believe that from there the disease was carried to the Western world. The Hebrews fleeing Egypt during the Exodus almost certainly had been contaminated. In 62 BC, after fighting in Egypt, Roman soldiers returned to Pompeii, spreading leprosy to Italy.

Leprosy peaked in the West during the Middle Ages. The pilgrims and advancing troops of the Crusades, from AD 1095 to 1272, spread the disease throughout Europe and the Middle East. In an attempt to control a disease they did not understand, rulers ordered that lepers be ostracized from the rest of society. Many cities built asylums, which were special houses where lepers were forced to live together. An estimated 19,000 "leper houses" were built in Europe.

Victims of leprosy who were not confined to leper houses were forced to wear a cape with a yellow cross sewn on to identify them. They also were forced to carry a wooden clapper or a bell to warn anyone who might approach. Lepers were forbidden to marry. In some cities, they were considered "dead to society," and death rites, like funerals, were held for them. Most likely, an exaggerated fear of leprosy caused people with other skin diseases to be called lepers and cast out from society as well.

Leprosy does not discriminate; even members of royalty were affected. But the risk of infection greatly increased in the poorest neighborhoods of the cities. People were crowded together in small homes with no running water. They washed infrequently. They shared beds to keep warm. Waste was disposed of in open sewers that ran along the streets. Poor nutrition weakened people's resistance to infection. These conditions created perfect breeding grounds for leprosy. These same conditions also fueled the Black Plague, a fast-spreading, deadly disease that terrorized much of European society in the 1340s.

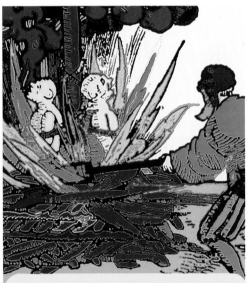

In the past, those thought to have caused outbreaks of disease were dealt with harshly. This painting portrays people executing suspected plague spreaders by burning them at the stake.

The Crusades were holy wars fought by European Christians to take Jerusalem and the surrounding areas from Muslims. The word "crusade" comes from the Latin *crux*, which means "cross." Crusaders wore a red cloth cross sewn onto their clothing to show that they were soldiers of Christ.

The First Crusade (1095–1099) began when Pope Urban II spoke at the Council of Clermont in France. He said that Jerusalem and the Holy Land should be controlled only by Christians. As a result, thousands of pilgrim-soldiers set out, crying *Deus vult*, or "God wills it." In July 1099, this First Crusade was successful in taking Jerusalem from the Muslims. But the success was short-lived.

The Muslims fought back. The Second Crusade (1147–1149) was launched by King Louis VII of France and King Conrad III of Germany with little success. The Muslims regained control of Jerusalem in 1187. The Third Crusade (1189–1192) was launched. Crusaders set out from France and England, but they did not even reach Jerusalem. The Fourth Crusade, begun in 1202, captured Constantinople, what is now Istanbul in Turkey, in 1204.

While the Crusades enabled pilgrims to encounter other cultures and share advances in science and medicine, disease was also shared. Because they were tired from their long journeys and weakened by poor nutrition, the pilgrims made perfect targets for the bacteria that caused leprosy. Since the symptoms of leprosy take so long to develop, the crusaders would not have known that they were infected. As they traveled, they spread their disease throughout Europe, finally taking it to their homes in England, France, Germany, Italy, and beyond.

An End to the Spread of Leprosy in Europe

Scientists believe that bubonic plague, also known as the Black Plague and the Black Death, began around 1346 in Mongolia. Fleas carried the disease, infecting millions of rodents, especially rats. These rats scurried through people's homes in search of food, leaving disease-infected fleas behind them. When the fleas bit people, the people became ill.

The disease was carried across Asia to Europe on the furs sold by traders, the clothing worn by travelers, and the rats that lived on ships. News of the millions of deaths that the plague caused reached Europe before the disease. It arrived in Italy in 1347 on a ship returning from Crimea, a peninsula that extends into the Black Sea. Rats from the ship carried fleas and infection to rats living near the

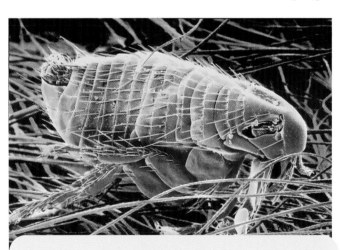

Fleas spread the bubonic plague and other diseases.

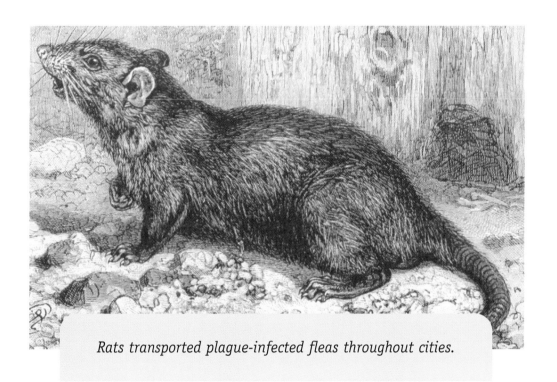

Rats transported plague-infected fleas throughout cities.

docks. Plague spread to the city, fueled further by sailors who had already been infected. People were terrified of being infected because they knew the plague led to a horrible death. The bacteria entered the human body from a flea or rat bite or by inhalation. Inside the body, it quickly spread to the lymph nodes, which became enlarged and filled with pus. Traveling through the bloodstream, the bacteria attacked the liver, spleen, and brain, sometimes causing dementia that led people to believe Satan possessed them. In the majority of cases, death occurred in just a few days.

No one knew then what caused bubonic plague or how to stop it. People tried to protect themselves by keeping travelers out of their cities. Wealthy landowners pulled up their drawbridges and sealed their gates, hiding from the peasants left to fend for themselves. Groups of people accused of spreading the Black Death were even murdered.

In 1666, much of London was destroyed by the Great Fire. The thatched roofs of London's homes, which had made perfect breeding grounds for fleas, fueled the fire, causing it to burn out of control. Although the Great Fire devastated London, it also helped stop the Black Death. The rat population declined. The tile and slate that were used to rebuild roofs did not offer homes to fleas. But the damage had been done. One-quarter to one-half of the population of Europe had died—estimated at nearly 75 million people.

When the plague was over, leprosy also began to die out in Europe. Although no one is sure why this happened, several explanations are possible. So many people died of the plague—nearly half the population of Europe—that the cities became less crowded. Once people were no longer packed into small spaces, infections did not spread as easily. It is also possible that those who survived the plague had very strong immune systems. Their bodies were able to fight off other diseases, like leprosy, as well. In addition, perhaps the people who would have been the most likely to get leprosy had already died from the plague.

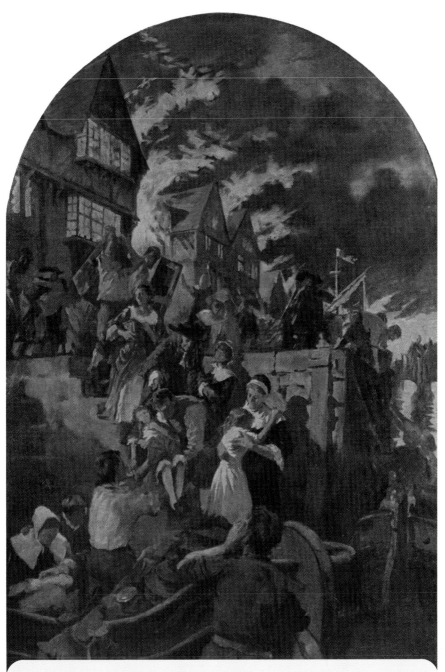

This painting by Forbes Stanhope depicts the Great Fire of London, which devastated the city but helped stop the Black Death.

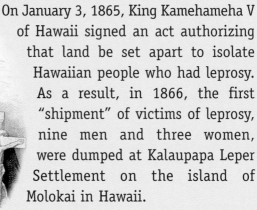

Father Damien

On January 3, 1865, King Kamehameha V of Hawaii signed an act authorizing that land be set apart to isolate Hawaiian people who had leprosy. As a result, in 1866, the first "shipment" of victims of leprosy, nine men and three women, were dumped at Kalaupapa Leper Settlement on the island of Molokai in Hawaii.

Horrible stories were told of new arrivals being forced to jump from the ship and swim for their lives. Rather than dock the ship and risk the infection they so gravely feared, the ship's crew would throw crates of supplies into the sea and rely on the incoming tide to carry them to shore. Conditions at the settlement were grim. Because there were no houses or buildings of any kind, the victims lived in caves or shelters that they built of rocks or tree limbs and dried leaves. There were no doctors, no hospitals—no treatment of any kind.

These conditions continued for seven years, until the arrival of Belgian-born Father Damien de Veuster in 1873. Under his guidance, homes and churches were built. He also arranged for medical services and funding from the government in Honolulu. Unfortunately, Father Damien himself contracted leprosy in 1888. The considerable publicity that this caused fueled the fear that the disease was highly contagious and uncontrollable.

The Kalaupapa leprosy settlement continued in operation until the 1940s, when the use of multidrug therapy treatments stopped the spread of the disease. In 1969, Hawaii's isolation laws were abolished. In 1980, President Jimmy Carter signed a law establishing Kalaupapa as a national historical park. It is still home to former patients who have chosen to stay.

The spread of tuberculosis (TB) in Europe also helped stop leprosy. The bacteria that cause leprosy are very similar to those that cause tuberculosis. People who have had TB and recovered seem to be immune to leprosy. The reverse also seems to be true. In areas where large numbers of people are infected with tuberculosis, leprosy is not likely to be a problem. And victims of leprosy are unlikely to have tuberculosis.

Leprosy gradually disappeared in Europe and by the end of the seventeenth century was very rare. At the same time that it declined in Europe, however, it was spreading to the European colonies in Africa. Also, Spanish conquistadors and other explorers brought the infection to North and South America. The slave trade contributed to the spread of leprosy in the United States.

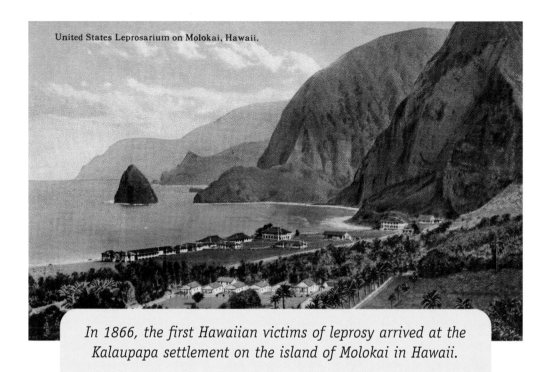

United States Leprosarium on Molokai, Hawaii.

In 1866, the first Hawaiian victims of leprosy arrived at the Kalaupapa settlement on the island of Molokai in Hawaii.

In the United States, leprosy became endemic in Texas, Louisiana, and Hawaii; a large number of people infected with the disease lived in these areas. As a result, two "settlements" for isolating patients with leprosy were established. In 1866, the first leprosy victims arrived at the Kalaupapa settlement on the island of Molokai in Hawaii. In 1894, the first patients were brought by barge from New Orleans to an abandoned plantation in Carville, Louisiana.

Unlike Kalaupapa, which existed primarily as a dumping ground for leprosy victims, Carville became a research center. It was there, in the early 1940s, that the Miracle at Carville (further explained in

A cousin of leprosy, tuberculosis (TB) is caused by tubercle bacilli, bacteria from the same genus, *Mycobacterium*, as leprosy. Just as they are able to defeat leprosy, the immune systems of many people are able to fight off TB, and the people may never know that they were infected. Like leprosy bacteria, tuberculosis bacteria can lie dormant in the body for a long time before symptoms of active tuberculosis appear.

The most common form of active TB, pulmonary tuberculosis, eats away the tissue of the lungs. The bacteria reach the lungs when small droplets coughed up by a person infected with active TB are inhaled. As the lungs are destroyed, the infected area fills with pus. The walls of the blood vessels that carry oxygen from the lungs are destroyed. The infected person will begin to cough up blood. Untreated TB will continue to eat away parts of the body, eventually causing uncontrolled internal bleeding that usually leads to death.

Other symptoms of TB include fatigue, loss of weight and appetite, night sweats, and fever. The disease progresses slowly so that it seems to be consuming the body. For this reason, tuberculosis was commonly referred to as consumption.

(continued on page 30)

chapter 3) occurred. It was discovered that sulfone drugs, like dapsone, could cure leprosy. Soon, a multiple drug therapy would be developed that would eliminate leprosy from much of the world.

(continued from page 29)

Finding a cure for TB was difficult. Researchers faced many of the same challenges as they did with leprosy. The bacteria that cause TB were identified by Robert Koch in 1882. But a drug that would successfully treat the disease was not produced until 1943, when Albert Schatz found that streptomycin killed tuberculosis bacteria.

Streptomycin produced dramatic results. Patients improved immediately, regaining their strength. Their lungs began to heal. But there were also problems. Some people were allergic to streptomycin and could not take it. Also, the TB bacteria became resistant, and patients who thought they were cured found their TB returning.

Like leprosy, tuberculosis requires a combination of drugs to completely defeat it. This multidrug therapy has greatly reduced the number of TB cases worldwide. However, in 1990, a strain that is resistant to four of the major TB drugs appeared in New York City. Researchers must continue to work to find new ways to control this stubborn disease.

THE SEARCH FOR A CURE

For centuries, leprosy remained one of the most mysterious and frightening diseases in the world. No one understood what caused it. Many people believed that it could not be cured because it was a curse from God.

Now we know that leprosy is an infectious disease caused by *M. leprae* bacteria. Bacteria are tiny, living organisms that can be seen only under a microscope. Thirty trillion bacteria of average size would weigh only one ounce. Until the microscope was invented in the late seventeenth century, scientists did not know bacteria existed. Once they could look through the microscope's lens to this hidden world, scientists found bacteria everywhere: on rotting leaves, inside an animal's mouth, even in a human stomach. Some 2,000 species of bacteria have been identified.

The rod-shaped bacteria that cause leprosy belong to a family of germs that includes the bacteria that cause tuberculosis. Most people, perhaps as much as 90 percent of the population, are naturally immune to leprosy. Their bodies are able to identify the leprosy bacteria as an invading germ, or antigen, defend against it, and kill it.

The body's first defense against invasion is the skin, the body's protective covering. Unless it has been cut, healthy skin keeps germs out. The body's fluids, such as tears and sweat, also help wash away bacteria. If antigens succeed in breaking through these defenses, special fighting cells, called macrophages, meet them, absorb them, and kill them. A battle takes place in the body, pitting bad cells against good cells. This causes inflammation.

Within most people, macrophages destroy the leprosy bacteria. These people never know that they were invaded and

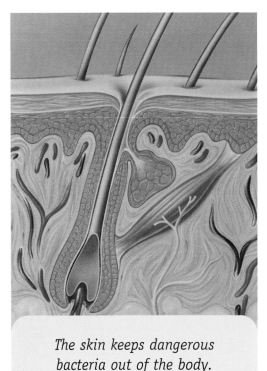

The skin keeps dangerous bacteria out of the body.

were in danger of becoming sick. In others, the macrophages are unable to kill the leprosy germs and instead carry them throughout the body, actually giving them a place to grow. Riding inside macrophages, the leprosy bacteria arrive at the Schwann cells, the outermost nerve cells of the body and the bacteria's favorite environment. Once in the body, leprosy bacteria grow very slowly, taking twelve to fourteen days for one cell to become two.

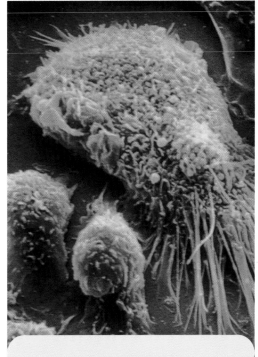

This is a microscopic photograph of a macrophage attacking a foreign body.

Hansen's Disease

In the early 1800s, the leprosy bacteria remained a mystery. Most doctors agreed with Daniel Danielssen that leprosy was hereditary. One man, Gerhard Henrick Armauer Hansen, thought differently. He thought that leprosy was contagious and was caused by a microorganism, an organism that could be seen only with a microscope. Hansen spent a year examining samples of diseased tissue from leprosy patients. He was looking for something that existed in all these samples but was not found in healthy tissue. On February 28, 1873, Hansen noticed tiny rods that he had not seen before. He checked many more samples and found the rods in all of them.

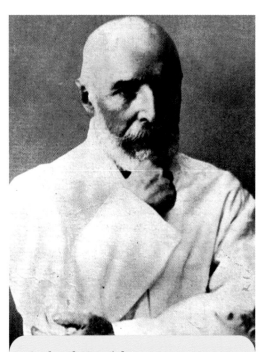

Gerhard Henrick Armauer Hansen was the first to find the bacteria that caused leprosy in humans.

Hansen thought he had found the cause of leprosy, but he still needed to test his theory. He injected animals with this new bacteria, but the animals failed to get sick. What Hansen did not know was that most animals cannot contract leprosy. Hansen was the first scientist to discover the bacteria that cause leprosy in humans, but he could not prove that these bacteria were the ones to blame.

Eventually, most doctors accepted Hansen's idea that leprosy is contagious. But no one was able to find a cure because they could not get the bacteria to grow outside of the human body. The bacteria would not grow in other animals or in a laboratory. It was almost impossible to test drugs to see if they would work against leprosy.

The first leprosy drugs were eventually tested on patients at the Carville leprosy research center. The patients volunteered for the studies because they were desperate to find a better treatment or a cure for their disease.

Treatment

Before the 1940s, leprosy was treated with a thick, badly smelling oil (called chaulmoogra) made from the nuts of the hydnocarpus, or kalaw, tree. According to legend, centuries ago a Burmese king who was suffering from leprosy was told by the gods to eat the kalaw fruit. After eating the fruit, he was cured. In many modern cases, the oil did kill *M. leprae*, but it was not always effective, and the side effects were unpleasant. If swallowed, the oil caused stomachaches. When injected, it caused painful sores on the skin. But at the time, it was the only treatment available.

On November 30, 1894, seven victims of leprosy were hidden on a coal barge and brought from New Orleans to an abandoned sugarcane plantation along the Mississippi River. For two years, the patients lived under the care of a resident doctor. On April 27, 1896, four sisters from the Daughters of Charity order arrived to provide nursing and household care at what became known as the Louisiana Leper Home. The promise of a safe place to live, considered by many to be a miracle, had occurred.

But it was a miracle with limits. Although no laws were ever passed in the United States requiring the isolation of leprosy patients, many states still sent people to Carville, usually by force. Some were brought in chains. Others arrived hidden in coffins because they feared an angry mob would attack them. Once inside, they no longer had the choice to leave. An on-site jail was ready for those caught trying to escape.

Over the years, conditions at Carville improved, largely as a result of the work of the residents. Rules forbidding marriage were dropped. On February 1, 1921, following the purchase of the plantation by the state of Louisiana, the National Leprosarium at Carville was established.

Carville became a research center as well as a hospital. Most patients were treated with chaulmoogra oil, the only known treatment for leprosy. But in the early 1940s, Dr. Guy Faget began experimenting with promin, a drug used to treat tuberculosis. Since the bacteria that cause leprosy and tuberculosis are similar, he thought perhaps the same drug would work with leprosy.

At the time, the only way to test whether promin would work was to experiment on humans. Many patients volunteered for the study because they wanted so badly to cure their leprosy. At first, promin did not seem to work. It made the patients so sick that many of them dropped out of the study. But after six months, those who had continued with the drug found that their symptoms began to disappear. Skin sores healed. Eyesight cleared. Doctors tested for the bacteria and found that the number of bacteria was greatly reduced. Promin was killing leprosy! It was a miracle!

Promin was not the final answer to the leprosy puzzle. Eventually, dapsone would replace it as the primary treatment. But the discovery of promin was the first step in the right direction toward the multidrug therapy that would allow doctors to call leprosy curable.

Then in the 1940s, Dr. Guy Faget, a doctor at Carville, tested an antibiotic drug called promin and, soon after, a similar compound called dapsone. Dapsone had been developed in 1908. It worked on tuberculosis, which is caused by bacteria very similar to *M. leprae*. Studies at Carville proved that dapsone was effective against leprosy, too. Until the early 1980s, leprosy patients would be treated daily with 100 milligrams of dapsone. The success of dapsone was short-lived, however. It worked very slowly, causing many patients to stop taking it.

More important, leprosy bacteria were able to become resistant to the drug. Further research, however, was still hampered by the inability to grow *M. leprae* in experimental animals.

Finally, in 1960, the leprosy bacteria were successfully grown in the footpads of mice. Research into new and more powerful drugs was possible. (The nine-banded armadillo, which has a primitive immune system and low body temperature, can also be infected with *M. leprae*.) Scientists developed multiple drug therapy (MDT), which includes dapsone, rifampicin, and clofazimine taken in combination. If leprosy is diagnosed early, MDT kills the bacteria before any serious nerve damage occurs. To be cured, patients must take these drugs for six to twenty-four months, depending on their symptoms.

MDT is vital because leprosy bacteria treated with only one drug soon develop resistance to it. Although the drug kills most of the bacteria, some of them survive the

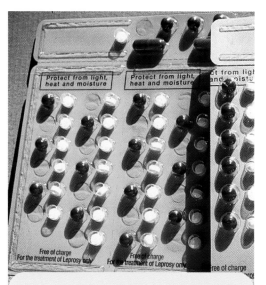

Taken in combination, dapsone, rifampicin, and clofazimine can cure leprosy if the disease is detected early.

treatment and continue to grow. Others mutate, or change, so that the drug cannot kill them. These bacteria can cause infection even though the patient is taking an antileprosy drug. If multiple drugs are used, however, the bacteria are unable to resist treatment, and they eventually die.

In 1980, the World Health Organization (WHO) formally recognized and used multiple drug therapy in its campaign to eliminate leprosy throughout the world.

Dr. Paul Brand

Most scientists concentrated their efforts on finding a way to kill *M. leprae*, the bacteria that cause leprosy. But Dr. Paul Brand, an orthopedic surgeon at a hospital in Vellore, India, looked for other ways to help. He was especially interested in the hand paralysis, or "claw hand," that leprosy caused. The upper joints of the fingers of patients with claw hand curled down toward their palms, as if they were starting to make a fist. These patients could clench their fists very tightly, but they could not open their fingers.

Brand began his research by examining the bodies of leprosy patients who had died. He discovered that in 80 percent of the patients, the ulnar nerve that ran along the outside of the arm was swollen with leprosy bacteria at the elbow and wrist. The muscles and tendons controlled by this nerve were paralyzed. But nerves that ran deeper through the arm were not damaged. The muscles that they controlled were healthy. Brand thought he might be able to correct the paralysis by moving tendons controlled by healthy nerves and muscles to the paralyzed part of the hand.

Leprosy paralyzes the muscles and tendons controlled by the ulnar nerve, resulting in "claw hand."

Brand performed a procedure on the thumb of his first patient. He cut a tendon that had been attached to the patient's ring finger and reattached it to the patient's thumb. But when the bandages were removed three weeks later, the patient was able to move his thumb only slightly. Brand was disappointed at first. He had hoped the thumb would move normally right away.

The problem was not with the surgery, however. It was in the patient's brain. The brain thought the tendon was still attached to the ring finger. When the patient thought "move my thumb," the brain sent the movement message to the paralyzed tendons. The thumb did not respond. Brand told the patient to try to move his ring finger. When the patient thought "move my ring finger," the brain sent the movement message to the tendons that were now attached to the thumb. The thumb moved!

After the first success, Brand moved other tendons. In each case, the patient needed to retrain his or her brain to send the correct movement signals to the tendons in the fingers. Once that happened, the patient had full use of his or her hands.

Brand worried about another serious problem for leprosy patients, too. Most had dangerous foot ulcers. Although Brand cleaned and rebandaged the sores on his patients' feet, they would not heal. Then one day, Brand watched a patient walk away from the hospital. The patient did not limp; because he did not feel pain, he walked normally, putting pressure on the infected ulcers with every step. Brand developed a plaster cast similar to the ones used to keep broken bones stable while they heal. When patients wore the casts on their feet, the ulcers were protected and healed.

Brand made another contribution to the care of leprosy patients. After surgery had given patients the use of their hands, Brand wanted to protect them. Although the fingers moved, they still did not feel pain. Some patients injured their hands accidentally or while working. Others found a more puzzling problem.

Sometimes, patients would wake up in the morning and find that their fingers were cut and bleeding. They could not explain their injuries. Finally, one man discovered a rat had chewed his hand during the night. Because the man could not feel pain, he did not wake up and chase the rat away. After that, Brand sent each of his patients home from the hospital with a cat.

In 1966, after twenty years in India, Brand moved to the leprosy hospital in Carville, Louisiana. He continued to work with leprosy patients, helping them avoid injury and healing them when injuries occurred.

4

WINNING THE BATTLE

In 1991, the World Health Organization outlined its goal to eliminate leprosy as a public health problem by 2000. To reach that goal, the number of leprosy cases would need to be reduced to less than one case per 10,000 people living in any country. While progress was made toward the goal, leprosy was not totally eliminated by 2000. Battles have been won in the fight against leprosy, but the war is not over.

In 1985, 122 countries were considered to be endemic. In these countries, large numbers of leprosy cases were always present. By the beginning of 2000, ninety-eight of these countries had reached the elimination goal. Around the world, leprosy has been reduced by 86 percent. More than 10 million patients had been cured by MDT by the end of 1999.

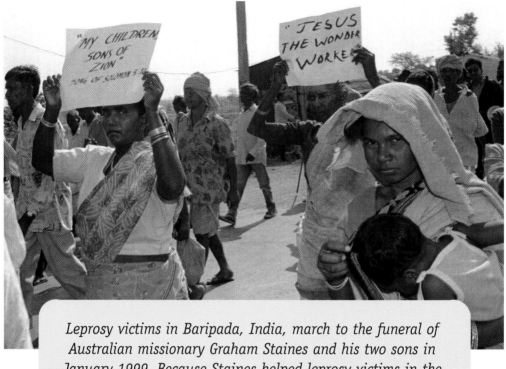

Leprosy victims in Baripada, India, march to the funeral of Australian missionary Graham Staines and his two sons in January 1999. Because Staines helped leprosy victims in the area, a group of radicals burned his family alive while they slept.

Leprosy remains a public health problem in twenty-four countries around the world, however. In 1999, the greatest number of leprosy cases worldwide, 67 percent, was in India. WHO knew of approximately 495,000 people in India with leprosy in 1999. Brazil, Indonesia, and Myanmar also have large numbers of cases. Eighty percent of the leprosy cases in Latin America were in Brazil. Myanmar had the largest concentration of cases, with nearly six cases per 10,000 people. Most of the other countries where leprosy is still endemic are in Africa.

Treating leprosy in Africa has been a big challenge for WHO. Other problems in African countries are more immediate. The AIDS epidemic, which kills thousands of people each year, has turned the focus away from leprosy. Health care resources are needed to treat AIDS and deadly tropical diseases. Also, many countries in Africa are involved in civil wars. People have been forced out of their homes and live in refugee camps, where they are unable to grow food or take care of livestock. Starvation and malnutrition are huge problems. In addition, doctors and nurses cannot physically get to sick patients because the dirt roads are often blocked by soldiers, and hospitals and clinics are far apart. It is difficult to get medicine to the people who need it. Under these conditions, treating leprosy is not as important as keeping people safe or finding food for them.

Although India is not at war, treating leprosy there is still difficult. Most people who have leprosy are members of the "untouchable" caste (class) and are still thought by many to be unclean. Some people believe that victims of leprosy have the disease as punishment for sins they committed in previous lives.

Fortunately, not everyone in India believes that victims of leprosy are unclean. Some hospitals and clinics are specifically devoted to caring for leprosy

India has more leprosy cases than any other country. Poverty, overpopulation, and poor sanitation and health care contribute to this problem. But India's caste system, which divides people into strict social classes, makes the situation there unique.

India's society is divided into groups, called castes, and each person is born into one of them. The main castes, called varnas, were developed about 1000–800 BC. The highest varna was the Brahmin. These men served as priests. Second, the Kshatriya, were warriors or political rulers. Members of the third varna, the Vaisya, were traders and farmers. The fourth, called Shudra, were artisans, builders, and laborers. Within these four varnas, more specific castes were ranked based on the "purity" of their work. For example, since gold was ranked as more pure than wood, goldsmiths ranked higher than carpenters.

A fifth caste developed later, the Panchama, or untouchable caste. Members of this group were forced to work in jobs considered unclean. Members of other castes had to avoid contact with untouchables or risk becoming unclean themselves.

Rules were designed to keep the castes "pure," or separate. For example, marriage between members of different castes was forbidden. Today, these rules have relaxed and Indian society is becoming more integrated.

The caste system is closely tied to the Hindu religion. In India, nearly 85 percent of the population is Hindu. One of the most important Hindu beliefs is in a kind of reincarnation called transmigration of souls. This belief, also called samsara, holds that a man's caste at birth, length of life, and experiences throughout life are directly related to the kind of person he was in a previous life. In other words, a Brahmin who enjoys a happy life is being rewarded for his good actions in a previous life.

The reverse would also be true. A man who suffers and is a member of the untouchable caste must have lived a horrible life previously. He is being punished for his sins.

In India, most people who suffer from leprosy belong to the untouchable class. This sometimes makes treatment difficult. Some people think that victims of leprosy deserve their disease. Also, rules of the caste system say that members of higher castes may not touch an untouchable. This can make it hard to find enough people who are willing to treat leprosy victims in India. Health care workers must help everyone understand that leprosy is a disease and not a punishment.

Treating all the people in India who have leprosy would be difficult because there are not enough health care workers. Transportation outside of the cities is primitive. People need to be trained to effectively administer multidrug therapy. But the caste system, which causes some people to believe that victims of leprosy have brought their suffering on themselves, makes the situation in India uniquely challenging.

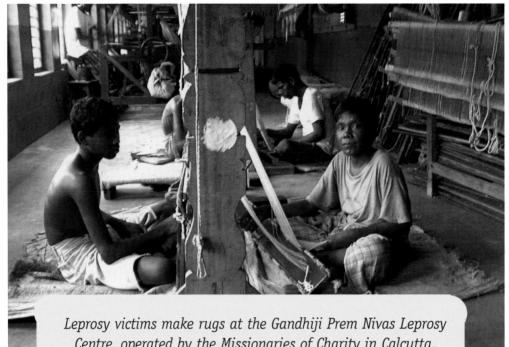

Leprosy victims make rugs at the Gandhiji Prem Nivas Leprosy Centre, operated by the Missionaries of Charity in Calcutta, India. The center helps those suffering from leprosy.

patients. One of the most famous, Shantinagar, was begun by Mother Teresa and the Missionaries of Charity. In addition to health care, people at Shantinagar are given jobs and treated with love and respect.

But many leprosy patients in India do not find their way to a hospital or clinic. This creates difficulties for WHO in fighting the disease. In order to reach everyone who has leprosy, WHO needs to train local people to provide the treatment. But some people think that treating untouchables is a waste of time. They do not believe that untouchables can be cured of their disease.

Even with trained people, treating leprosy in India and other poorer countries is a very hard job. MDT requires that three drugs be taken over a minimum six-month period. The drugs are taken in different amounts that change during the course of treatment. Patients must be monitored to be sure that they are taking the drugs correctly. If they do not take the right amount of each drug every day, the treatment will not work.

Keeping people on their treatment schedules is difficult because many untouchables do not have homes. In cities, they may live on the street and move around a lot. Health care workers cannot keep track of them from one day to the next. Most leprosy victims are poor. They do not have money for food, so they certainly cannot afford to buy a clock or watch. Without knowing what time it is, they do not know when it is time to take their medicine. They cannot always know when they took their last dose. For MDT to work, the combination of drugs must be taken regularly.

For MDT to be most effective, it should be started as early as possible, as soon as leprosy is diagnosed. But people living in poverty, especially in areas far from cities, cannot get to a doctor to find out why they are sick. The leprosy bacteria get a strong hold before the patient can get any medicine.

Also, because there is still a high degree of prejudice against leprosy, many people try to hide their disease. When the only symptom is a small skin rash, no one will notice. Instead of seeing a doctor to find out what is causing their rash, they may avoid doctors so no one will find out that they have leprosy and call them "unclean."

Even more advanced stages of leprosy can be cured by MDT. Unfortunately, though, while the bacteria will be killed, not all the disabilities will be corrected. For example, cartilage around the nose that has been eaten away by disease will not grow back. Injuries to hands and feet that occurred because a patient did not feel pain are not the direct result of leprosy. They may need additional treatment, such as surgery.

With multiple drug therapy, leprosy can be cured. But the treatment is complicated and lengthy. Social conditions in some countries present challenges that have made MDT less effective than WHO had hoped. Researchers continue to look for a single drug that could be used against leprosy. They are also working to develop a vaccine.

5

THE FUTURE OF LEPROSY

The World Health Organization is still working to eliminate leprosy worldwide. In most countries, this goal has been achieved. For example, according to the Hansen's Disease Center in Carville, in the United States in 1995 there were only 6,000 registered cases of leprosy. In the United States, approximately 170 new cases are reported annually, of which 85 percent to 90 percent are among immigrants from countries where leprosy is a larger problem.

While this is relatively good news, scientists warn that leprosy should not be ignored. Most doctors in the United States have little knowledge of leprosy because it is so uncommon there. Also, the focus of American medical research has been shifted away from leprosy to diseases like AIDS that present a more immediate danger and affect larger numbers of people.

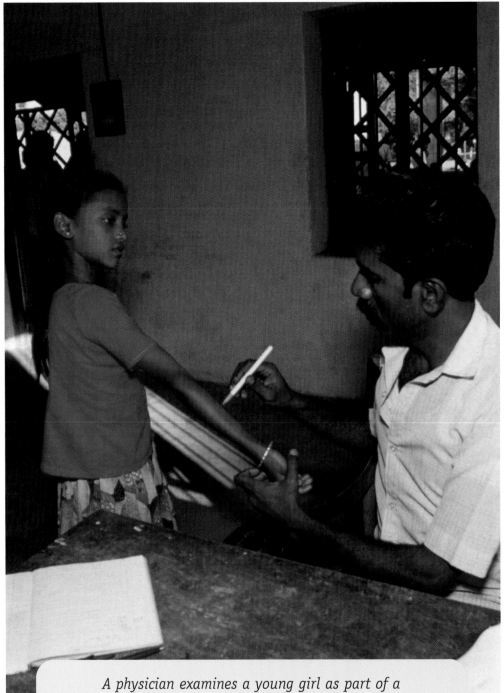

A physician examines a young girl as part of a leprosy study in Polambakkam, India.

It is true that leprosy is no longer a large problem in the United States. But in many poorer countries, it continues to cause pain and suffering to great numbers of people. These countries cannot afford to spend money on medical research. Qualified experts are not available to them. They must rely on countries like the United States to continue working to solve the problems of leprosy around the world.

In 1997, the World Health Organization reported that progress has been made in leprosy research. Two new drugs, minocycline and clarithromycin, have shown promising results. These drugs are being tested in an attempt to cut down the number of doses patients are required to take. In addition, researchers continue tests to develop a vaccine.

Managing patient care is one of WHO's biggest challenges. Multiple drug therapy is provided free of charge to all patients. Getting the drugs to everyone who needs them and monitoring patients to be sure they take the drugs is difficult in remote areas. To reach patients living in difficult-to-access areas, a special program, Special Action Projects for the Elimination of Leprosy (SAPEL) is used. SAPEL's first objective is to find patients with leprosy who live in difficult areas. SAPEL provides the MDT drugs and teaches people how to take them effectively. It also teaches other members of the community to help monitor patients and recognize future leprosy cases that may develop. And SAPEL helps the community understand that people being treated for leprosy can still work and go to school; they do not need to be sent away or avoided.

If MDT services are not extended to difficult-to-access areas, the goal of eliminating leprosy will be hard to reach. In addition, WHO worries that patients who do not understand MDT and are not monitored carefully may take the drugs incorrectly. This can cause new strains of resistant leprosy. Patients may take the drugs for a while, feel better quickly, and think they are cured. They will then suffer a relapse, which is the return of their symptoms. Or, they may become confused and take the MDT drugs in the wrong combination. It is especially important not to take rifampicin by itself. Rifampicin-resistant leprosy would be very difficult to fight.

Finally, it is important to continue research in new and better ways to help people who have been disabled by leprosy. While the focus now is on elimination, in the future higher priority can be given to improving people's lives after their leprosy has been cured.

New cases of leprosy will continue to occur in small numbers, even when the elimination goal has been reached, as people who were infected several years earlier report symptoms. Factors beyond the control of WHO, like civil war, will continue to challenge efforts to reach leprosy patients. But today leprosy, or Hansen's disease, is totally curable. Successful elimination is on the horizon.

GLOSSARY

antigen   An invading germ.

asylum   Sequestered place where lepers were forced to live.

bacteria   Microscopic organisms, some of which cause infectious diseases.

contagious disease   Disease that can be transmitted from person to person; also called infectious disease.

endemic disease   Disease that is widespread in a particular area or among a particular group of people.

immune system   Body's natural system of defense against disease.

infection   Invasion of the body by disease-causing bacteria or the condition that results from the invasion.

inflammation Pain, swelling, and redness in an area of the body that has been injured or infected.

macrophages Cells that protect the body against infection.

Mycobacterium leprae (*M. leprae*) Bacteria that cause leprosy.

pilgrim One who journeys to a sacred place.

psoriasis Skin disease that causes white, scaly patches.

resistance The body's ability to successfully fight off disease.

tuberculosis Highly infectious disease caused by bacteria similar to *Mycobacterium leprae*.

FOR MORE INFORMATION

In the United States

American Leprosy Foundation
11600 Nebel Street
Rockville, MD 20852
(301) 984-1336
Web site: http://users.erols.com/lwm-alf

American Leprosy Missions
1 ALM Way
Greenville, SC 29601
(800) 543-3135
Web site: http://www.leprosy.org

Centers for Disease Control and Prevention (CDC)
1600 Clifton Road
Atlanta, GA 30333
(404) 639-3311
Web site: http://www.cdc.gov

National Institute of Allergy and Infectious Disease
Office of Communications and Public Liaison
31 Center Drive MSC 2520
Building 31, Room 7A-50
Bethesda, MD 20892-2520
(301) 496-5717
Web site: http://www.niaid.nih.gov

International

INFOLEP Leprosy Information Services
Netherlands Leprosy Relief
P.O. Box 95005
1090 HA Amsterdam
The Netherlands
31 (0) 20 595 0530
Web site: http://infolep.antenna.nl

International Leprosy Association
Global Project on the History of Leprosy
22 Tiverton Road
24 Eversholt Street
London NW10 3HL
United Kingdom
44 (0) 20 8969 4830
Web site: http://www.leprosyhistory.org

The World Health Organization (WHO) and Pan
      American Health Organization
525 Twenty-third Street NW
Washington, DC 20037
(202) 974-3000
Web site: http://www.who.org
Web site: http://www.paho.org

FOR FURTHER READING

Brand, Paul, and Philip Yancey. *Pain: The Gift Nobody Wants*. New York: HarperCollins, 1993.

Farrell, Jeanette. *Invisible Enemies: Stories of Infectious Disease*. New York: Farrar, Straus & Giroux, 1998.

Garrett, Laurie. *The Coming Plague: Newly Emerging Diseases in a World Out of Balance*. New York: Farrar, Straus & Giroux, 1994.

Johnson, Linda Carlson. *Mother Teresa: Protector of the Sick*. New York: Blackbirch Press, 1991.

Karlen, Arno. *Man and Microbes: Disease and Plagues in History and Modern Times*. New York: Simon & Schuster, 1996.

Martin, Betty. *Miracle at Carville*. New York: Doubleday, 1950.

Ramen, Fred. *Tuberculosis*. New York: The Rosen Publishing Group, Inc., 2001.

INDEX

CREDITS

About the Author

Karen Donnelly, a freelance writer, lives in Connecticut with her husband, David, and daughters, Cathy and Colleen. She has written several books for the Rosen Publishing Group, including *Coping with Dyslexia*, *Everything You Need to Know About Lyme Disease*, and *Coolcareers.com: Hardware Engineer*.

Photo Credits

Cover and chapter interior photos © Dr. Kari Lounatmaal/Science Photo Library/Photo Researchers; pp. 4, 11, 40 © Paul A. Souders/Corbis; p. 6 © Corbis; pp. 10, 32 © Custom Medical; p. 12 © Christine Osborne/Photo Researchers; p. 13, 34 © Science Photo Library/Photo Researchers; pp. 18, 25 © Hulton/Archive; p. 20 © Sheila Terry/Science Photo Library/Photo Researchers; p. 22 © Dr. Tony Brain/Science Photo Library/Photo Researchers; p. 23 © Photo Researchers; p. 26 © North Wind; p. 28 © Lake County Museum/Corbis; p. 33 © Manfred Kage/Peter Arnold; p. 38 © A. Crump, TDR/Science Photo Library/Photo Researchers; p. 44 © AP/Wide World Photos; p. 48 © AP/*Lincoln Journal Star*; p. 52 © Janet Wishnetsky/Corbis.

Series Design

Evelyn Horovicz

Layout

Les Kanturek